NO GALLBLADDER DIET COOKBOOK FOR BEGINNERS

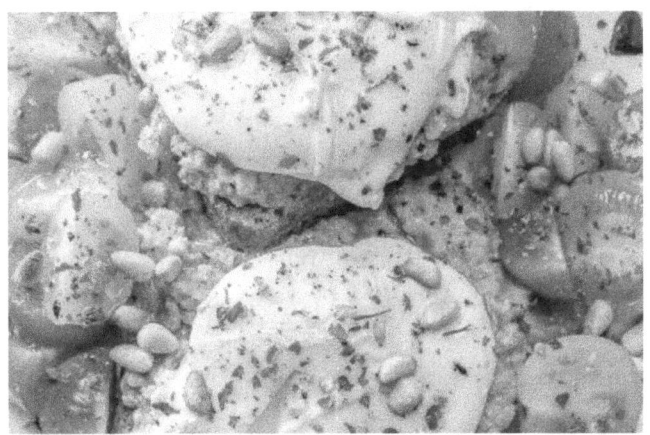

The Complete Guide to Flavorful and Nourishing Recipes To Balance Your Metabolism After Gallbladder Removal, With 30 Day Meal Plan.

Sharon D. Stacy

Table of Content

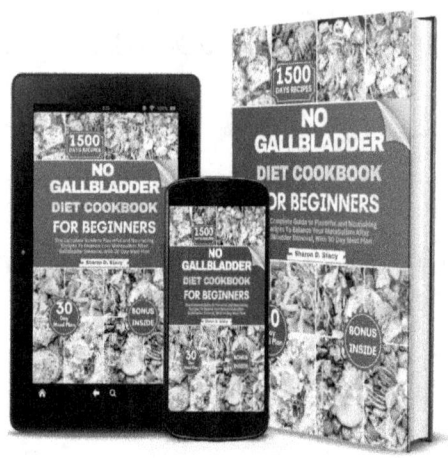

NO GALLBLADDER DIET COOKBOOK FOR BEGINNERS

How to Use This Book

1. Introduction and Understanding Gallbladder Health: Begin by reading the introduction to gain a basic understanding of the importance of gallbladder health and how it impacts your overall well-being.

2. Common Issues After Gallbladder Removal: Familiarize yourself with common challenges individuals face after gallbladder removal surgery. This section will help you anticipate potential issues and understand why certain dietary adjustments are necessary.

3. Principles of a Gallbladder-Friendly Diet: Dive into the principles of a gallbladder-friendly diet, including what foods to include and avoid. Understanding these guidelines will empower you to make informed decisions about your dietary choices.

4. **Recipes:** Explore the wide variety of delicious and nutritious recipes tailored specifically for individuals without a gallbladder. Each recipe is designed with your health in mind, incorporating ingredients that support digestion and minimize discomfort.

5. **Meal Plans:** Utilize the provided 30-day meal plan as a guide for incorporating these recipes into your daily routine. This structured approach will help you stay on track and ensure a balanced diet over time.

6. **Nutritional Information:** Refer to the nutritional information provided for each recipe to understand its macronutrient content and make informed choices based on your dietary needs and goals.

7. **Shopping List:** Use the included shopping list to streamline your grocery shopping experience. This comprehensive list will ensure you have all the necessary ingredients on hand to whip up delicious meals without hassle.

8. **Notes/Progress Report:** Keep track of your progress, thoughts, and any modifications you make to the recipes in the Notes/Progress Report section. This will help you personalize your experience and fine-tune your dietary habits over time.

9. **Conclusion and Final Thoughts:** Reflect on your journey and celebrate your successes. The conclusion offers words of encouragement and support as you continue on your path towards better health and well-being.

By following these steps and utilizing the resources provided in this cookbook, you'll be well-equipped to navigate life without a gallbladder and enjoy a fulfilling, satisfying diet that supports your overall health and vitality.

INTRODUCTION

Ever wonder what it would be like to live without a gallbladder? Maybe you had surgery to remove it recently, and you're now navigating an uncertain world of nutrition. Many think that avoiding fatty foods completely is the best way to go about life after gallbladder removal. What if I told you, though, that this widely held notion is not totally true?

Let's delve into the intricacies of life without a gallbladder. The liver produces bile, which the gallbladder stores and releases, which is essential for the breakdown of fats. In the absence of this tiny but powerful organ, the breakdown of fats can be interfered with, causing pain and digestive issues.

Now imagine living a life free from the constant fear that a meal will bring you pain or distress. Imagine being able to eat tasty, filling meals without worrying about any negative effects on your digestive system. This is where the "No Gallbladder Diet Cookbook For Beginners" comes in.

You will learn a great deal about navigating life without a gallbladder with assurance and ease by reading this in-depth guide. This book covers everything, from realizing the significance of dietary adjustments to picking up useful advice for organizing and preparing meals.

I understand the challenges and frustrations that come with adjusting to life post-gallbladder surgery. This cookbook was created with great care to be your go-to guide when it comes to restoring the health of your digestive system. Say goodbye to discomfort and guesswork and hello to a future full of satisfying meals that are customized to meet your specific needs. Allow this book to be your go-to resource for dietary advice following gallbladder removal, helping you live a longer, happier life.

CHAPTER 1

Understanding Gallbladder

The gallbladder is a small, pear-shaped organ located just beneath the liver. Its main function is to store and concentrate bile, a digestive fluid produced by the liver, and release it into the small intestine to aid in the digestion of fats.

When you eat a meal containing fats, the gallbladder contracts and releases bile into the small intestine via the bile duct. Bile helps emulsify fats, breaking them down into smaller droplets that can be more easily digested and absorbed by the body. This process is essential for the absorption of fat-soluble vitamins (A, D, E, and K) and the digestion of dietary fats.

While the gallbladder plays an important role in the digestion of fats, it is not considered a vital organ, meaning you can live without it. In some cases, people may need to have their gallbladder removed due to gallstones, inflammation (cholecystitis), or other gallbladder-related conditions. Cholecystectomy is the surgical term for this procedure.

After gallbladder removal, bile flows directly from the liver into the small intestine instead of being stored and concentrated in the gallbladder. While most people can live a normal, healthy life without a gallbladder, some may experience digestive symptoms such as diarrhea, bloating, or difficulty digesting fatty foods. Adopting a low-fat diet and making dietary adjustments can help manage these symptoms and promote better digestion post-surgery.

Thriving Without a Gallbladder

Thriving without a gallbladder is absolutely possible with some adjustments to your lifestyle and diet. While the gallbladder plays a role in fat digestion, its absence doesn't mean you can't live a healthy, fulfilling life. Here's how you can thrive without a gallbladder:

1. **Gradual dietary adjustments:** After gallbladder removal, you may find that certain foods, especially high-fat ones, can trigger digestive discomfort. Start by gradually reintroducing foods into your diet and noting how your body reacts. Focus on smaller, more frequent meals and opt for lean proteins, whole grains, fruits, and vegetables.

2.   **Balanced, low-fat diet:** Aim to consume a well-balanced diet that is low in fat, particularly saturated and trans fats. Instead, choose healthy fats such as those found in avocados, nuts, seeds, and fatty fish like salmon. Incorporate plenty of fiber-rich foods to support digestion and promote regularity.

3.   **Mindful eating:** Pay attention to how your body responds to different foods. To keep track of your meals and any related symptoms, keep a food journal. This can help you identify trigger foods and make informed choices about what to include in your diet.

4.   **Stay hydrated:** Drink plenty of water throughout the day to support digestion and prevent dehydration. Adequate hydration can also help to soften stools and alleviate constipation, which may occur post-gallbladder removal.

5.   **Regular physical activity:** Engage in regular exercise to promote overall health and well-being. Physical activity can aid digestion, boost metabolism, and help maintain a healthy weight, which is important for managing digestive symptoms and overall health.

6.   **Consult with healthcare professionals:** If you experience persistent digestive issues or have concerns about your diet post-gallbladder removal, don't hesitate to seek guidance from healthcare professionals. A registered dietitian or healthcare provider can provide personalized recommendations and support to help you thrive without a gallbladder.

By making mindful dietary choices, staying active, and seeking support when needed, you can thrive without a gallbladder and enjoy a healthy, fulfilling lifestyle.

Common Issues After Gallbladder Removal

After gallbladder removal surgery, also known as cholecystectomy, some individuals may experience certain digestive issues as their body adjusts to the absence of the gallbladder and changes in bile flow. These common issues may include:

1.　　Diarrhea or loose stools: Without the gallbladder to store and concentrate bile, bile acids may flow more continuously into the intestines, leading to diarrhea or loose stools in some individuals. This is often temporary but can persist for some people.

2.　　Bloating and gas: Changes in bile flow and digestion can sometimes lead to increased gas production and bloating, especially after consuming high-fat or large meals.

3.   **Difficulty digesting fatty foods:** Since the gallbladder's role is to store bile and release it when needed to digest fats, some individuals may have difficulty digesting fatty foods after its removal. This may result in diarrhea, bloating, or discomfort.

4.   **Increased risk of bile reflux:** Without the gallbladder to regulate bile release, some individuals may experience bile reflux, where bile flows backward into the stomach, causing irritation and discomfort.

5.   **Digestive discomfort or pain:** Some individuals may experience ongoing or intermittent abdominal pain or discomfort after gallbladder removal, which can be related to

various factors such as scar tissue formation or residual bile duct stones.

6. **Post-cholecystectomy syndrome:** In rare cases, individuals may develop post-cholecystectomy syndrome, characterized by persistent abdominal pain, bloating, and digestive issues after gallbladder removal. This may be due to factors such as bile duct injury, sphincter of Oddi dysfunction, or other gastrointestinal conditions.

It's important to note that not everyone experiences these issues after gallbladder removal, and many people adjust well to life without a gallbladder. However, if you're experiencing persistent or severe digestive symptoms after gallbladder surgery, it's essential to consult with your healthcare provider for evaluation and appropriate management. Dietary adjustments, medications, and other treatments may help alleviate symptoms and improve your quality of life post-cholecystectomy.

Principles of Gallbladder Friendly Diet

A gallbladder-friendly diet focuses on reducing the intake of certain foods that may trigger digestive discomfort or symptoms after gallbladder removal. Here are some principles to follow:

1.   Low-fat foods: Limiting your intake of high-fat foods can help reduce the risk of digestive issues post-gallbladder removal. Opt for lean proteins such as poultry, fish, and legumes, and choose low-fat or fat-free dairy products.

2.   Healthy fats: While you should reduce your intake of saturated and trans fats, incorporate healthy fats into your diet, such as those found in avocados, nuts, seeds, and olive

oil. These fats are easier to digest and less likely to cause digestive discomfort.

3. **High-fiber foods:** Include plenty of fiber-rich foods in your diet, such as fruits, vegetables, whole grains, and legumes. Fiber helps promote regularity and prevent constipation, which can be common after gallbladder removal.

4. **Moderate portions:** Avoid overeating or consuming large meals, as this can put strain on your digestive system and increase the risk of symptoms. Instead, aim for smaller, more frequent meals throughout the day to support digestion.

5. **Hydration:** Drink plenty of water throughout the day to stay hydrated and support digestion. Adequate hydration can help prevent

constipation and promote the smooth passage of food through the digestive tract.

6. **Avoid trigger foods:** Identify and avoid foods that may trigger digestive symptoms or discomfort, such as spicy foods, fried foods, high-fat meats, processed foods, and carbonated beverages. Everyone's triggers may vary, so pay attention to how your body responds to different foods.

7. **Slowly reintroduce foods:** After gallbladder removal, gradually reintroduce foods into your diet and monitor how your body reacts. Start with bland, easily digestible foods and gradually expand your diet as tolerated.

8. **Mindful eating:** Practice mindful eating by chewing your food thoroughly, eating slowly, and paying attention to your body's hunger and fullness cues. In addition to

lowering the chance of digestive problems, this can help avoid overeating.

9. Consult with a healthcare professional: If you're unsure about which foods to include or avoid in your gallbladder-friendly diet, or if you're experiencing persistent digestive symptoms, seek individualized advice and assistance from a registered dietitian or other healthcare provider. They can help you develop a tailored eating plan to meet your individual needs and promote digestive health post-gallbladder removal.

Foods to Avoid

After gallbladder surgery, it's important to avoid certain foods that may trigger digestive discomfort or exacerbate symptoms. Here are some foods to avoid:

1. **High-fat foods:** Foods that are high in fat can be difficult to digest after gallbladder removal and may lead to symptoms such as diarrhea, bloating, or abdominal pain. Avoid fried foods, fatty cuts of meat, processed snacks, and creamy or cheesy dishes.

2. **Spicy foods:** Spicy foods can irritate the digestive tract and may exacerbate symptoms such as heartburn or acid reflux. Avoid dishes seasoned with hot peppers, chili powder, or other spicy ingredients.

3. **Greasy or fried foods:** Greasy or fried foods are high in fat and can be hard to digest, particularly after gallbladder surgery. Steer clear of deep-fried foods, fast food, and dishes cooked in heavy oils or butter.

4. **Processed foods:** Processed foods often contain additives, preservatives, and unhealthy fats that can aggravate digestive issues. Limit your intake of processed snacks, packaged meals, and convenience foods.

5. **High-cholesterol foods:** High-cholesterol foods can contribute to the formation of bile stones and may increase the risk of complications post-gallbladder surgery. Avoid foods high in cholesterol, such as organ meats, egg yolks, and full-fat dairy products.

6.   **Gas-producing foods:** Certain foods can cause gas and bloating, which may be uncomfortable after gallbladder surgery. Eat less of the foods that cause gas, such as beans, cabbage, onions, and carbonated drinks.

7.   **Raw vegetables and fruits with skins:** Raw vegetables and fruits with tough skins or seeds may be difficult to digest, particularly in the immediate aftermath of gallbladder surgery. Opt for cooked or peeled vegetables and fruits to reduce the risk of digestive discomfort.

8.   **Alcohol and caffeine:** Alcohol and caffeine can irritate the digestive tract and may worsen symptoms such as acid reflux or diarrhea. Drinks high in caffeine, like soda, coffee, and tea, should be consumed in moderation.

9.   **Large meals:** Eating large meals can put strain on the digestive system and may increase the risk of symptoms such as bloating or abdominal pain. Instead, opt for smaller, more frequent meals throughout the day to support digestion.

10.   **Spicy and acidic foods:** Spicy and acidic foods, such as citrus fruits, tomatoes, and vinegar-based dressings, may exacerbate symptoms such as heartburn or acid reflux. Limit your intake of these foods to reduce the risk of discomfort.

It's important to listen to your body and avoid any foods that cause digestive discomfort or exacerbate symptoms after gallbladder surgery.

Gradually reintroduce foods into your diet and pay attention to how your body responds. If you're unsure about which foods to avoid or include in your post-surgery diet, consult with a healthcare professional or registered dietitian for personalized guidance and support.

Shopping List

1. Lean proteins:

- Skinless poultry (chicken, turkey)

- Fish (salmon, trout, cod)

- Lean cuts of beef or pork (loin, sirloin)

- Eggs

- Tofu or tempeh (for vegetarian options)

2. Low-fat dairy products:

- Skim or low-fat milk

- Plain yogurt (unsweetened)

- Cottage cheese (low-fat or fat-free)

- Reduced-fat cheese (mozzarella, feta)

3. Healthy fats:

- Avocados

- Nuts and seeds (almonds, walnuts, chia seeds)

- Olive oil or avocado oil

- Flaxseed oil

4. High-fiber foods:
  - Fresh fruits (apples, berries, pears)
  - Vegetables (leafy greens, broccoli, carrots)
  - Whole grains (quinoa, brown rice, oats)
  - Legumes (beans, lentils)

5. Whole grains and cereals:
  - Whole wheat bread or wraps
  - Whole grain pasta
  - Brown rice
  - Oatmeal or whole grain cereal

6. Fresh produce:
  - Leafy greens (spinach, kale, lettuce)
  - Cruciferous vegetables (broccoli, cauliflower, Brussels sprouts)
  - Colorful vegetables (bell peppers, tomatoes, cucumbers)
  - Fresh fruits (apples, oranges, bananas)

7. Herbs, spices, and flavorings:

- Fresh herbs (parsley, cilantro, basil)
- Garlic and ginger (fresh or powdered)
- Low-sodium vegetable or chicken broth
- Vinegars (apple cider vinegar, balsamic vinegar)

8. Beverages:

- Water
- Herbal teas (peppermint, chamomile)
- Low-acid fruit juices (apple, pear)

9. Snacks and treats:

- Rice cakes
- Air-popped popcorn
- Whole grain crackers
- Unsweetened dried fruits (apricots, raisins)

10. Miscellaneous:

- Low-sodium soy sauce or tamari

- Mustard and low-fat mayonnaise

- Natural sweeteners (honey, maple syrup)

11. Protein alternatives:

- Plant-based protein sources like tofu, tempeh, and edamame

- Canned beans (black beans, kidney beans, chickpeas)

12. Dairy alternatives:

- Unsweetened almond milk, oat milk or even soy milk

- Dairy-free yogurt (made from soy, coconut, or almond)

13. Cooking oils:

- Canola oil

- Grapeseed oil

- Coconut oil (in moderation)

14. Condiments and dressings:

- Low-fat salad dressings (vinaigrettes)

- Reduced-sodium soy sauce or tamari

- Hot sauce (choose low-sodium varieties)

15. Frozen foods:

- Frozen fruits (berries, mango chunks, pineapple)

- Frozen vegetables (mixed vegetables, spinach, broccoli)

- Frozen fish fillets or shrimp

16. Baking ingredients:

- Whole wheat flour or almond flour

- Baking powder and baking soda

- Unsweetened applesauce (as a baking substitute for oil or butter)

17. Nuts and seeds:

- Pumpkin seeds
- Sunflower seeds
- Cashews (unsalted)

18. Beverages:

- Unsweetened coconut water
- Green tea
- Sparkling water (plain or flavored with natural fruit essences)

19. Grains and pasta alternatives:

- Quinoa
- Buckwheat
- Whole grain couscous

20. Sweeteners and flavor enhancers:

- Stevia
- Monk fruit sweetener
- Vanilla extract (unsweetened)

Remember to plan your meals ahead of time and use your shopping list as a guide to ensure you have everything you need for healthy and gallbladder-friendly meals throughout the week. Customize your shopping list based on your personal preferences and dietary needs. Additionally, it's important to read food labels carefully and choose low-fat, low-sodium, and minimally processed options whenever possible. Happy shopping and happy cooking!

CHAPTER 2

Breakfast Recipes

1. Creamy Oatmeal with Fresh Berries

Ingredients:

- ½ cup rolled oats

- 1 cup water or milk

- ¼ cup fresh berries (such as strawberries, blueberries, or raspberries)

- 1 tablespoon maple syrup or honey

- Pinch of cinnamon (optional)

Preparation:

1. In a small saucepan, bring the water or milk to a boil.

2. Stir in the rolled oats and reduce the heat to low. Cook for 5-7 minutes, stirring occasionally, until the oats are creamy and tender.

3. Remove from heat and let the oatmeal cool slightly.

4. Transfer the oatmeal to a bowl and top with fresh berries, honey or maple syrup, and a pinch of cinnamon, if desired.

5. Serve warm and enjoy!

Nutritional Value (per serving):

- Calories: 200

- Protein: 5g

- Carbohydrates: 35g

- Fat: 4g

- Fiber: 5g

Cooking Time: 10 minutes

Notes:

_____

_____

_____

_____

_____

_____

Progress Report:

_____

_____

_____

_____

_____

_____

2. Scrambled Eggs with Spinach and Feta

Ingredients:

- 2 large eggs
- 1 cup fresh spinach, chopped
- 2 tablespoons crumbled feta cheese
- Salt and pepper, to taste
- Cooking spray or olive oil

Preparation:

1. Whisk the eggs in a bowl until well beaten. Season with salt and pepper.

2. Ensure you heat a non-stick skillet over medium heat and lightly coat with cooking spray or olive oil.

3. Add the chopped spinach to the skillet and cook for 1-2 minutes until wilted.

4. Pour the beaten eggs over the spinach and cook, stirring occasionally, until the eggs are scrambled and cooked through.

5. Sprinkle the scrambled eggs with crumbled feta cheese and serve hot.

Nutritional Value (per serving):

- Calories: 220

- Protein: 14g

- Carbohydrates: 3g

- Fat: 17g

- Fiber: 1g

Cooking Time: 5 minutes

Notes:

_____

_____

_____

_____

_____

_____

Progress Report:

_____

_____

_____

_____

_____

_____

3. Banana Walnut Pancakes

Ingredients:

- 1 ripe banana, mashed
- 2 large eggs
- ¼ cup chopped walnuts
- ½ teaspoon ground cinnamon
- Cooking spray or butter (for cooking)

Preparation:

1. Mash the ripe banana in a bowl until it's smooth. Add the eggs, chopped walnuts, and ground cinnamon, and mix until well combined.

2. Apply a thin layer of cooking spray or butter to a non-stick skillet or griddle that is heated over medium heat.

3. Pour ¼ cup of the pancake batter onto the skillet and cook for 2-3 minutes, until bubbles form on the surface.

4. Flip the pancake and cook for an additional 1-2 minutes, until golden brown and cooked through.

5. Repeat with the remaining batter to make additional pancakes.

6. Serve the pancakes warm with your favorite toppings, such as maple syrup or Greek yogurt.

Nutritional Value (per serving, 2 pancakes):
- Calories: 320
- Protein: 14g
- Carbohydrates: 20g
- Fat: 22g
- Fiber: 4g

Cooking Time: 10 minutes

Notes:

_____

_____

_____

_____

_____

_____

Progress Report:

_____

_____

_____

_____

_____

_____

4.   Greek Yogurt Parfait

Ingredients:

- 1 cup Greek yogurt (plain, unsweetened)
- ½ cup granola (low-fat, low-sugar)
- ½ cup mixed fresh berries (such as strawberries, blueberries, raspberries)
- 1 tablespoon maple syrup or honey

Preparation:

1. In a serving glass or bowl, layer Greek yogurt, granola, and mixed fresh berries.

2. Repeat the layers until all ingredients are used, ending with a layer of berries on top.

3. Drizzle with honey or maple syrup, if desired.

4. When ready to eat, serve straight away or store in the refrigerator.

Nutritional Value (per serving):

- Calories: 300

- Protein: 20g

- Carbohydrates: 35g

- Fat: 10g

- Fiber: 6g

Cooking Time: 5 minutes

Notes:

_____

_____

_____

_____

_____

_____

Progress Report:

_____

_____

_____

_____

_____

_____

5. Apple Cinnamon Quinoa Porridge

Ingredients:

- ½ cup quinoa, rinsed
- 1 cup water or milk
- 1 small apple, diced
- ½ teaspoon ground cinnamon
- 1 tablespoon maple syrup or honey
- Chopped nuts or dried fruit (optional, for garnish)

Preparation:

1. In a small saucepan, combine the quinoa and water or milk. Bring to a boil, then reduce the heat to low and simmer for 15-20 minutes, until the quinoa is cooked and the liquid is absorbed.

2. Stir in the diced apple and ground cinnamon, and cook for an additional 2-3 minutes until the apple is softened.

3. Remove from heat and stir in honey or maple syrup, if desired.

4. Serve the quinoa porridge warm, garnished with chopped nuts or dried fruit if desired.

Nutritional Value (per serving):

- Calories: 280

- Protein: 8g

- Carbohydrates: 50g

- Fat: 5g

- Fiber: 6g

Cooking Time: 25 minutes

Notes:

_____

_____

_____

_____

_____

_____

Progress Report:

_____

_____

_____

_____

_____

_____

6. Avocado Toast with Poached Eggs

Ingredients:

- 2 slices whole grain bread

- 1 ripe avocado

- 2 large eggs

- Salt and pepper, to taste

- Red pepper flakes (optional, for garnish)

Preparation:

1. Toast the slices of whole grain bread until golden brown and crispy.

2. Meanwhile, slice the ripe avocado and mash it with a fork until smooth. Season with salt and pepper to make it tasty.

3. Fill a small saucepan with water and bring to a simmer over medium heat. Break the eggs into individual small bowls or ramekins.

4. Gently slide the eggs into the simmering water and cook for 3-4 minutes, until the whites are set but the yolks are still runny.

5. Remove the poached eggs from the water with a slotted spoon and drain on a paper towel.

6. Spread the mashed avocado evenly onto the toasted bread slices.

7. Top each avocado toast with a poached egg and sprinkle with red pepper flakes, if desired.

8. Serve immediately, while the eggs are still warm.

Nutritional Value (per serving, 1 slice of toast with 1 poached egg):

- Calories: 220

- Protein: 12g

- Carbohydrates: 15g

- Fat: 13g

- Fiber: 6g

Cooking Time: 10 minutes

Notes:

_____

_____

_____

_____

_____

_____

Progress Report:

_____

_____

_____

_____

_____

_____

7. Sweet Potato Hash with Turkey Sausage

Ingredients:

- 1 large sweet potato, diced
- 2 links turkey sausage, sliced
- ½ onion, diced
- 1 bell pepper, diced
- 2 cloves garlic, minced
- 1 teaspoon smoked paprika
- Salt and pepper, to taste
- Olive oil (for cooking)

Preparation:

1. Ensure you heat a large skillet over medium heat and add a drizzle of olive oil.
2. Add the diced sweet potato to the skillet and cook for 5-7 minutes, until lightly browned and tender.

3. Add the sliced turkey sausage, diced onion, bell pepper, and minced garlic to the skillet. Cook for an additional 5-7 minutes, until the vegetables are softened and the sausage is cooked through.

4. Season the hash with smoked paprika, salt, and pepper to taste, and cook for another 1-2 minutes.

5. Serve the sweet potato hash hot, garnished with fresh herbs if desired.

Nutritional Value (per serving):

- Calories: 300
- Protein: 15g
- Carbohydrates: 30g
- Fat: 15g
- Fiber: 6g

Cooking Time: 20 minutes

Notes:

_____

_____

_____

_____

_____

_____

Progress Report:

_____

_____

_____

_____

_____

_____

8.   Blueberry Chia Pudding

Ingredients:

- ¼ cup chia seeds
- 1 cup unsweetened almond milk (or any other milk of choice)
- ½ cup fresh or frozen blueberries
- 1 tablespoon maple syrup or honey
- ½ teaspoon vanilla extract

Preparation:

1. In a mixing bowl, combine the chia seeds, almond milk, honey or maple syrup (if using), and vanilla extract. Stir well to combine.

2. Gently fold in the fresh or frozen blueberries.

3. Cover the bowl and refrigerate for at least 4 hours or overnight, until the chia seeds have absorbed the liquid and formed a pudding-like consistency.

4. Stir the chia pudding before serving and adjust sweetness to taste, if necessary.

5. Serve the blueberry chia pudding chilled, garnished with additional blueberries or a drizzle of honey, if desired.

Nutritional Value (per serving):

- Calories: 200

- Protein: 6g

- Carbohydrates: 25g

- Fat: 8g

- Fiber: 10g

Cooking Time: 5 minutes (plus chilling time)

Notes:

_____

_____

_____

_____

_____

_____

Progress Report:

_____

_____

_____

_____

_____

_____

9. Cottage Cheese and Fruit Bowl

Ingredients:

- ½ cup low-fat cottage cheese
- ½ cup mixed fresh fruit (such as sliced strawberries, pineapple chunks, and grapes)
- 1 tablespoon of chopped nuts (like walnuts or almonds)
- Drizzle of honey or maple syrup (optional)

Preparation:

1. In a serving bowl, spoon the low-fat cottage cheese.

2. Top with mixed fresh fruit and chopped nuts.

3. Drizzle with honey or maple syrup, if desired.

4. Serve the cottage cheese and fruit bowl immediately.

Nutritional Value (per serving):

- Calories: 180
- Protein: 12g
- Carbohydrates: 20g
- Fat: 7g
- Fiber: 3g

Cooking Time: 5 minutes

Notes:

_____

_____

_____

_____

_____

_____

Progress Report:

_____

_____

_____

_____

_____

_____

10. Zucchini and Carrot Fritters

- 1 large zucchini, grated
- 1 large carrot, grated
- 2 eggs
- ¼ cup whole wheat flour
- 2 tablespoons chopped fresh herbs (such as parsley or dill)
- Salt and pepper, to taste
- Olive oil (for cooking)

Preparation:

1. In a large mixing bowl, combine the grated zucchini, grated carrot, eggs, whole wheat flour, chopped fresh herbs, salt, and pepper. Mix until well combined.

2. A non-stick skillet should be heated over medium heat and add a drizzle of olive oil.

3. Drop spoonfuls of the fritter batter onto the skillet and flatten with the back of a spoon.

4. Cook the fritters for 3-4 minutes on each side, until golden brown and cooked through.

5. Remove the fritters from the skillet and drain on a paper towel.

6. Serve the zucchini and carrot fritters hot, garnished with a dollop of Greek yogurt or a squeeze of lemon juice if desired.

Nutritional Value (per serving, 2 fritters):

- Calories: 200
- Protein: 8g
- Carbohydrates: 15g
- Fat: 10g
- Fiber: 5g

Cooking Time: 15 minutes

Notes:

_____

_____

_____

_____

_____

_____

Progress Report:

_____

_____

_____

_____

_____

_____

CHAPTER 2

Lunch Recipes

1. Baked Lemon Herb Salmon

Ingredients:

- 4 salmon fillets (4-6 ounces each)

- 2 tablespoons olive oil

- 2 tablespoons fresh lemon juice

- 2 cloves garlic, minced

- 1 tablespoon chopped fresh herbs (such as dill, parsley, or thyme)

- Salt and pepper, to taste

- Lemon slices (for garnish)

Preparation:

1. Preheat the oven to 375°F (190°C). Ensure you line a baking sheet with parchment paper or foil.

2. After the baking sheet is ready, put the salmon fillets on it.

3. In a small bowl, whisk together the olive oil, lemon juice, minced garlic, chopped fresh herbs, salt, and pepper.

4. Drizzle the lemon herb mixture over the salmon fillets, coating them evenly.

5. Bake the salmon in the preheated oven for 12-15 minutes, until cooked through and flaky.

6. Remove from the oven and garnish with lemon slices before serving.

Nutritional Value (per serving):

- Calories: 300

- Protein: 25g

- Carbohydrates: 2g

- Fat: 20g
- Fiber: 0g

Cooking Time: 15 minutes

Notes:

_____

_____

_____

_____

_____

_____

Progress Report:

_____

_____

_____

_____

_____

_____

2. Grilled Shrimp Skewers

Ingredients:

- 1 pound of large, peeled and deveined shrimp
- 2 tablespoons olive oil
- 2 cloves garlic, minced
- 1 tablespoon of freshly chopped herbs, like cilantro or parsley
- Salt and pepper, to taste
- Lemon wedges (for serving)

Preparation:

1. Preheat the grill to medium-high heat.

2. Thread the shrimp onto skewers, leaving a little space between each shrimp.

3. In a small bowl, whisk together the olive oil, minced garlic, chopped fresh herbs, salt, and pepper.

4. Brush the garlic herb mixture onto the shrimp skewers, coating them evenly.

5. Grill the shrimp skewers for 2-3 minutes per side, until pink and cooked through.

6. Remove from the grill and serve hot with lemon wedges on the side.

Nutritional Value (per serving):

- Calories: 200

- Protein: 25g

- Carbohydrates: 1g

- Fat: 10g

- Fiber: 0g

Cooking Time: 6 minutes

Notes:

_____

_____

_____

_____

_____

Progress Report:

_____

_____

_____

_____

_____

3. Baked Cod with Tomato and Basil

Ingredients:

- 4 cod fillets (4-6 ounces each)
- 2 cups cherry tomatoes, halved
- 2 cloves garlic, minced
- 2 tablespoons olive oil
- ¼ cup chopped fresh basil
- Salt and pepper, to taste
- Lemon wedges (for serving)

Preparation:

1. Preheat the oven to 375°F (190°C). Lightly grease a baking dish with olive oil.

2. After the baking dish is ready, put the cod fillets in it.

3. In a mixing bowl, combine the cherry tomatoes, minced garlic, olive oil, chopped fresh basil, salt, and pepper. Toss to coat.

4. Arrange the tomato mixture around the cod fillets in the baking dish.

5. Bake the cod in the preheated oven for 15-20 minutes, until the fish is opaque and flakes easily with a fork.

6. Remove from the oven and serve hot with lemon wedges on the side.

Nutritional Value (per serving):

- Calories: 250
- Protein: 30g
- Carbohydrates: 5g
- Fat: 12g
- Fiber: 1g

Cooking Time: 20 minutes

Notes:

_____

_____

_____

_____

_____

_____

Progress Report:

_____

_____

_____

_____

_____

_____

4. Lemon Garlic Butter Scallops

Ingredients:

- 1 pound sea scallops
- 2 tablespoons butter
- 2 cloves garlic, minced
- 2 tablespoons fresh lemon juice
- 1 tablespoon chopped fresh parsley
- Salt and pepper, to taste
- Lemon wedges (for serving)

Preparation:

1. Using paper towels, pat the scallops dry, then season with salt and pepper.

2. Heat a large skillet over medium-high heat and add the butter.

3. Once the butter is melted, add the minced garlic to the skillet and cook for 1 minute, until fragrant.

4. Add the scallops to the skillet in a single layer, making sure not to overcrowd the pan.

5. Cook the scallops for 2-3 minutes per side, until golden brown and cooked through.

6. Remove the skillet from heat and add the fresh lemon juice and chopped parsley, tossing to coat the scallops.

7. Serve the lemon garlic butter scallops hot with lemon wedges on the side.

Nutritional Value (per serving):

- Calories: 200

- Protein: 25g

- Carbohydrates: 4g

- Fat: 10g

- Fiber: 0g

Cooking Time: 6 minutes

Notes:

_____

_____

_____

_____

_____

_____

Progress Report:

_____

_____

_____

_____

_____

_____

5.   Salmon and Asparagus Foil Packet

Ingredients:

- 2 salmon fillets (4-6 ounces each)

- 1 bunch asparagus, trimmed

- 2 tablespoons olive oil

- 2 cloves garlic, minced

- 1 tablespoon fresh lemon juice

- Salt and pepper, to taste

- Lemon slices (for garnish)

Preparation:

1. Preheat the oven to 400°F (200°C).

2. Place each salmon fillet on a piece of aluminum foil large enough to wrap around it.

3. Arrange the trimmed asparagus spears around the salmon fillets.

4. In a small bowl, whisk together the olive oil, minced garlic, fresh lemon juice, salt, and pepper.

5. Drizzle the lemon garlic mixture over the salmon and asparagus, coating them evenly.

6. Fold the edges of the foil over the salmon and asparagus to create a packet, sealing tightly.

7. Place the foil packets on a baking sheet and bake in the preheated oven for 15-20 minutes, until the salmon is cooked through and the asparagus is tender.

8. Remove from the oven and garnish with lemon slices before serving.

Nutritional Value (per serving):

- Calories: 300

- Protein: 25g

- Carbohydrates: 5g

- Fat: 20g

- Fiber: 2g

Cooking Time: 20 minutes

Notes:

_____

_____

_____

_____

_____

_____

Progress Report:

_____

_____

_____

_____

_____

_____

6.   Lime Cilantro Shrimp Tacos

Ingredients:

- 1 pound shrimp, peeled and deveined

- 2 tablespoons olive oil

- 2 cloves garlic, minced

- 1 teaspoon ground cumin

- ½ teaspoon chili powder

- ¼ teaspoon cayenne pepper (optional)

- Juice of 2 limes

- ¼ cup chopped fresh cilantro

- Salt and pepper, to taste

- Corn tortillas (for serving)

- Toppings: shredded cabbage, diced avocado, salsa, lime wedges

Preparation:

1. In a mixing bowl, combine the shrimp, olive oil, minced garlic, ground cumin, chili powder,

cayenne pepper (if using), lime juice, chopped fresh cilantro, salt, and pepper. Toss to coat.

2. Heat a large skillet over medium-high heat and add the seasoned shrimp.

3. Cook the shrimp for 2-3 minutes per side, until pink and cooked through.

4. Use a microwave or a dry skillet to reheat the corn tortillas.

5. Fill each tortilla with cooked shrimp and your favorite toppings, such as shredded cabbage, diced avocado, salsa, and lime wedges.

6. Serve the lime cilantro shrimp tacos hot, with extra lime wedges on the side.

Nutritional Value (per serving):
- Calories: 250
- Protein: 25g
- Carbohydrates: 20g
- Fat: 10g
- Fiber: 5g

Cooking Time: 10 minutes

Notes:

_____

_____

_____

_____

_____

_____

Progress Report:

_____

_____

_____

_____

_____

_____

7. Baked Teriyaki Salmon

Ingredients:

- 4 salmon fillets (4-6 ounces each)
- ¼ cup low-sodium soy sauce or tamari
- 2 tablespoons honey or maple syrup
- 2 cloves garlic, minced
- 1 teaspoon grated ginger
- 1 tablespoon rice vinegar
- Sesame seeds (for garnish)
- Sliced green onions (for garnish)

Preparation:

1. Preheat the oven to 400°F (200°C). Ensure you line a baking sheet with parchment paper or foil.

2. In a small saucepan, combine the low-sodium soy sauce or tamari, honey or maple syrup, minced garlic, grated ginger, and rice vinegar.

Simmer for two to three minutes, or until slightly thickened, over medium heat.

3. Place the salmon fillets on the prepared baking sheet and brush with the teriyaki sauce, reserving some for serving.

4. Bake the salmon in the preheated oven for 12-15 minutes, until cooked through and flaky.

5. Remove from the oven and garnish with sesame seeds and sliced green onions.

6. Serve the baked teriyaki salmon hot, with extra sauce on the side.

Nutritional Value (per serving):

- Calories: 300

- Protein: 25g

- Carbohydrates: 10g

- Fat: 15g

- Fiber: 0g

Cooking Time: 15 minutes

Notes:

_____

_____

_____

_____

_____

_____

Progress Report:

_____

_____

_____

_____

_____

8. Broiled Lemon Pepper Haddock

Ingredients:

- 4 haddock fillets (4-6 ounces each)
- 2 tablespoons olive oil
- 2 cloves garlic, minced
- 1 teaspoon lemon zest
- 1 tablespoon fresh lemon juice
- 1 teaspoon ground black pepper
- Salt, to taste
- Lemon wedges (for serving)

Preparation:

1. Preheat the broiler in the oven.

2. Place the haddock fillets on a baking sheet lined with foil or parchment paper.

3. In a small bowl, whisk together the olive oil, minced garlic, lemon zest, lemon juice, ground black pepper, and salt.

4. Brush the lemon pepper mixture over the haddock fillets, coating them evenly.

5. Broil the haddock fillets in the preheated oven for 8-10 minutes, until cooked through and lightly browned on top.

6. Remove from the oven and serve hot with lemon wedges on the side.

Nutritional Value (per serving):

- Calories: 250

- Protein: 30g

- Carbohydrates: 2g

- Fat: 12g

- Fiber: 0g

Cooking Time: 10 minutes

Notes:

_____

_____

_____

_____

_____

_____

Progress Report:

_____

_____

_____

_____

_____

_____

9. Shrimp and Vegetable Stir Fry

Ingredients:

- 1 pound shrimp, peeled and deveined
- 2 cups mixed veggies (like bell peppers, broccoli, snap peas)
- 2 tablespoons olive oil
- 2 cloves garlic, minced
- 1 tablespoon grated ginger
- 2 tablespoons low-sodium soy sauce or tamari
- 1 tablespoon hoisin sauce
- 1 teaspoon sesame oil
- Cooked quinoa or brown rice
- Sesame seeds (for garnish)
- Sliced green onions (for garnish)

Preparation:

1. Heat a large skillet or wok over medium-high heat and add the olive oil.

2. Add the minced garlic and grated ginger to the skillet and cook for 1 minute, until fragrant.

3. Add the mixed vegetables to the skillet and stir-fry for 3-4 minutes, until crisp-tender.

4. Slide the veggies to one side of the skillet, then top with the shrimp.

5. Cook the shrimp for 2-3 minutes per side, until pink and cooked through.

6. Combine the shrimp and vegetables in the skillet and add the low-sodium soy sauce or tamari, hoisin sauce, and sesame oil. Stir to coat.

7. Serve the shrimp and vegetable stir-fry hot over cooked brown rice or quinoa, garnished with sesame seeds and sliced green onions.

Nutritional Value (per serving):

- Calories: 300

- Protein: 25g

- Carbohydrates: 20g

- Fat: 12g

- Fiber: 5g

Cooking Time: 10 minutes

Notes:

_____

_____

_____

_____

_____

_____

Progress Report:

_____

_____

_____

_____

_____

_____

10. Baked Garlic Herb Mussels

Ingredients:

- 2 pounds mussels, cleaned and debearded
- 4 cloves garlic, minced
- 2 tablespoons olive oil
- ¼ cup chopped fresh parsley
- ¼ cup dry white wine (optional)
- Salt and pepper, to taste
- Lemon wedges (for serving)

Preparation:

1. Preheat the oven to 425°F (220°C). Line a baking sheet with foil.

2. In a large mixing bowl, toss the cleaned mussels with minced garlic, olive oil, chopped fresh parsley, dry white wine (if using), salt, and pepper.

3. Transfer the seasoned mussels to the prepared baking sheet in a single layer.

4. Bake the mussels in the preheated oven for 10-12 minutes, until the shells have opened and the mussels are cooked through.

5. Remove from the oven and discard any unopened shells before serving.

6. Serve the baked garlic herb mussels hot with lemon wedges on the side.

Nutritional Value (per serving):

- Calories: 200
- Protein: 20g
- Carbohydrates: 5g
- Fat: 10g
- Fiber: 1g

Cooking Time: 12 minutes

Notes:

_____

_____

_____

_____

_____

_____

Progress Report:

_____

_____

_____

_____

_____

_____

CHAPTER 4

Dinner Recipes

1. Lemon Herb Grilled Chicken Breast

Ingredients:

- 4 skinless, boneless chicken breasts, weighing 4-6 ounces apiece
- 2 tablespoons olive oil
- 2 tablespoons fresh lemon juice
- 2 cloves garlic, minced
- 1 tablespoon chopped fresh herbs (such as rosemary, thyme, or oregano)
- Salt and pepper, to taste
- Lemon slices (for garnish)

Preparation:

1. In a bowl, whisk together olive oil, lemon juice, minced garlic, chopped fresh herbs, salt, and pepper.

2. Place chicken breasts in a shallow dish and pour the marinade over them, making sure they are evenly coated. For a minimum of half an hour and a maximum of four hours, marinate in the refrigerator.

3. Preheat grill to medium-high heat. After removing the chicken from the marinade, discard any extra marinade.

4. Grill chicken for 6-8 minutes per side, or until internal temperature reaches 165°F (74°C).

5. Take it from the grill and give it a few minutes to rest before serving.

6. Serve hot, garnished with lemon slices.

Nutritional Value (per serving):

- Calories: 250

- Protein: 30g

- Carbohydrates: 1g

- Fat: 14g

- Fiber: 0g

Cooking Time: 15 minutes

Notes:

_____

_____

_____

_____

_____

_____

Progress Report:

_____

_____

_____

_____

_____

_____

2. Herb Crusted Chicken Thighs

Ingredients:

- 4 boneless, skinless chicken thighs
- ¼ cup breadcrumbs
- 2 tablespoons grated Parmesan cheese
- 1 teaspoon of dried herbs, like thyme, basil, or oregano
- Salt and pepper, to taste
- 1 tablespoon olive oil

Preparation:

1. Preheat oven to 400°F (200°C). Line a baking sheet with parchment paper.

2. In a shallow dish, combine breadcrumbs, Parmesan cheese, dried herbs, salt, and pepper.

3. Brush chicken thighs with olive oil, then coat them with breadcrumb mixture, pressing gently to adhere.

4. Place chicken thighs on prepared baking sheet and bake for 25-30 minutes, or until golden brown and cooked through.

5. Remove from oven and let rest for a few minutes before serving.

Nutritional Value (per serving):

- Calories: 300
- Protein: 25g
- Carbohydrates: 5g
- Fat: 18g
- Fiber: 1g

Cooking Time: 30 minutes

Notes:

_____

_____

_____

_____

_____

_____

Progress Report:

_____

_____

_____

_____

_____

_____

3. Honey Mustard Glazed Turkey Breast

Ingredients:

- 1 turkey breast (about 2 pounds)
- ¼ cup Dijon mustard
- 2 tablespoons honey
- 1 tablespoon olive oil
- 2 cloves garlic, minced
- Salt and pepper, to taste
- Fresh herbs (for garnish)

Preparation:

1. Preheat oven to 375°F (190°C). Use foil or parchment paper to line a baking dish..

2. In a small bowl, whisk together Dijon mustard, honey, olive oil, minced garlic, salt, and pepper.

3. Place turkey breast in the prepared baking dish and brush with honey mustard mixture, covering it evenly.

4. Roast turkey breast in the preheated oven for 45-60 minutes, or until internal temperature reaches 165°F (74°C), basting occasionally with pan juices.

5. Before slicing, take out of the oven and give it a 10-minute rest.

6. Add some fresh herbs as a garnish and serve hot.

Nutritional Value (per serving):

- Calories: 250

- Protein: 30g

- Carbohydrates: 5g

- Fat: 10g

- Fiber: 0g

Cooking Time: 60 minutes

Notes:

_____

_____

_____

_____

_____

_____

Progress Report:

_____

_____

_____

_____

_____

_____

4. Zucchini Noodles with Pesto

Ingredients:

- 4 medium zucchini, spiralized
- ½ cup basil pesto
- ¼ cup grated Parmesan cheese
- Cherry tomatoes, halved (for garnish)
- Pine nuts (for garnish)

Preparation:

1. Heat a large skillet over medium heat. Add spiralized zucchini and cook for 2-3 minutes, until tender.

2. Remove skillet from heat and toss zucchini noodles with basil pesto until evenly coated.

3. Divide zucchini noodles among plates and sprinkle with grated Parmesan cheese.

4. Garnish with cherry tomatoes and pine nuts before serving.

Nutritional Value (per serving):

- Calories: 200
- Protein: 5g
- Carbohydrates: 10g
- Fat: 15g
- Fiber: 3g

Cooking Time: 5 minutes

Notes:

_____

_____

_____

_____

_____

_____

Progress Report:

_____

_____

_____

_____

_____

_____

5.   Creamy Mushroom Risotto

Ingredients:

- 1 cup Arborio rice

- 4 cups chicken or vegetable broth

- 2 tablespoons olive oil

- 1 onion, finely chopped

- 2 cloves garlic, minced

- 8 ounces mushrooms, sliced

- ¼ cup grated Parmesan cheese

- Salt and pepper, to taste

- Chopped fresh parsley (for garnish)

Preparation:

1. In a saucepan, heat chicken or vegetable broth over low heat until warm.

2. In a separate large skillet, heat olive oil over medium heat. Add chopped onion and minced garlic, and cook until softened.

3. Add sliced mushrooms to the skillet and cook until tender and browned.

4. Stir in Arborio rice and cook for 1-2 minutes, until lightly toasted.

5. Gradually add warm broth to the skillet, ½ cup at a time, stirring constantly until absorbed before adding more.

6. Continue adding broth and stirring until rice is creamy and tender, about 20-25 minutes.

7. Remove skillet from heat and stir in grated Parmesan cheese. Season with salt and pepper to make it tasty.

8. When ready to serve, garnish with freshly cut parsley.

Nutritional Value (per serving):

- Calories: 300

- Protein: 8g

- Carbohydrates: 40g

- Fat: 10g

- Fiber: 3g

Cooking Time: 30 minutes

Notes:

_____

_____

_____

_____

_____

_____

Progress Report:

_____

_____

_____

_____

_____

_____

6. Baked Eggplant Parmesan

- 1 large eggplant, sliced into rounds
- 1 cup marinara sauce
- 1 cup shredded mozzarella cheese
- ¼ cup grated Parmesan cheese
- ½ cup breadcrumbs
- 2 tablespoons chopped fresh basil
- Olive oil spray

Preparation:

1. Preheat oven to 375°F (190°C). Line a baking sheet with parchment paper.

2. Lay out the slices of eggplant on the baking sheet that has been prepared, and drizzle with a little olive oil.

3. Bake eggplant slices for 15 minutes, flipping halfway through, until tender.

4. Remove eggplant slices from oven and spread marinara sauce on each slice.

5. Sprinkle shredded mozzarella cheese and grated Parmesan cheese over the marinara sauce.

6. In a small bowl, combine breadcrumbs and chopped fresh basil. Sprinkle breadcrumb mixture over the cheese.

7. Return eggplant slices to the oven and bake for an additional 10-15 minutes, until cheese is melted and bubbly.

8. When ready to serve, remove from oven and allow it cool for a few minutes.

Nutritional Value (per serving):

- Calories: 250

- Protein: 10g

- Carbohydrates: 20g

- Fat: 15g

- Fiber: 5g

Cooking Time: 30 minutes

Notes:

_____

_____

_____

_____

_____

_____

Progress Report:

_____

_____

_____

_____

_____

_____

7. Cauliflower and Broccoli Bake

Ingredients:

- 1 head cauliflower, cut into florets
- 1 head broccoli, cut into florets
- 2 tablespoons olive oil
- 2 cloves garlic, minced
- ¼ cup grated Parmesan cheese
- Salt and pepper, to taste
- ¼ cup breadcrumbs
- 2 tablespoons chopped fresh parsley

Preparation:

1. Preheat oven to 375°F (190°C). Grease a baking dish with olive oil.

2. In a large mixing bowl, toss cauliflower and broccoli florets with olive oil, minced garlic, grated Parmesan cheese, salt, and pepper.

3. Transfer seasoned vegetables to the prepared baking dish and spread them out evenly.

4. In a small bowl, combine breadcrumbs and chopped fresh parsley. Sprinkle breadcrumb mixture over the vegetables.

5. Bake in the preheated oven for 25-30 minutes, until vegetables are tender and breadcrumbs are golden brown.

6. Remove from oven and let cool for a few minutes before serving.

Nutritional Value (per serving):

- Calories: 150
- Protein: 7g
- Carbohydrates: 15g
- Fat: 8g
- Fiber: 7g

Cooking Time: 30 minutes

Notes:

_____

_____

_____

_____

_____

_____

Progress Report:

_____

_____

_____

_____

_____

_____

8. Eggplant and Chickpea Curry

Ingredients:

- 1 large eggplant, diced
- 1 can chickpeas, drained and rinsed
- 1 onion, finely chopped
- 2 cloves garlic, minced
- 1 tablespoon curry powder
- 1 teaspoon ground cumin
- 1 teaspoon ground coriander
- ½ teaspoon turmeric
- 1 can coconut milk
- Salt and pepper, to taste
- Chopped fresh cilantro (for garnish)
- Cooked rice (for serving)

Preparation:

1. Heat olive oil in a large skillet or pot over medium heat. Add diced eggplant and cook until golden brown.

2. Add chopped onion and minced garlic to the skillet and cook until softened.

3. Stir in curry powder, ground cumin, ground coriander, and turmeric, and cook for 1 minute until fragrant.

4. Add drained chickpeas and coconut milk to the skillet, stirring to combine.

5. Simmer curry for 15-20 minutes, until eggplant is tender and flavors are well combined.

6. Season with salt and pepper to make it tasty.

7. Serve hot over cooked rice, garnished with chopped fresh cilantro.

Nutritional Value (per serving):

- Calories: 300

- Protein: 8g

- Carbohydrates: 25g

- Fat: 20g

- Fiber: 8g

Cooking Time: 30 minutes

Notes:

_____

_____

_____

_____

_____

_____

Progress Report:

_____

_____

_____

_____

_____

_____

9.   Ratatouille

Ingredients:

- 1 eggplant, diced

- 2 zucchini, diced

- 1 bell pepper, diced

- 1 onion, diced

- 2 cloves garlic, minced

- 2 tomatoes, diced

- 2 tablespoons olive oil

- 1 tablespoon tomato paste

- 1 teaspoon of dried herbs (like basil, thyme, or oregano)

- Salt and pepper, to taste

- Chopped fresh parsley (for garnish)

Preparation:

1. Heat olive oil in a large skillet or pot over medium heat. Add diced onion and minced garlic, and cook until softened.

2. Add diced eggplant, zucchini, bell pepper, and tomatoes to the skillet, stirring to combine.

3. Stir in tomato paste and dried herbs, and season with salt and pepper to taste.

4. Cover and simmer ratatouille for 20-25 minutes, stirring occasionally, until vegetables are tender.

5. Remove from heat and let cool for a few minutes before serving.

6. Before serving, garnish with freshly cut parsley.

Nutritional Value (per serving):

- Calories: 200

- Protein: 5g

- Carbohydrates: 25g

- Fat: 10g
- Fiber: 8g

Cooking Time: 30 minutes

Notes:

_____

_____

_____

_____

_____

_____

Progress Report:

_____

_____

_____

_____

_____

_____

10. Sweet Potato and Lentil Curry

Ingredients:

- 2 sweet potatoes, diced
- 1 cup dried lentils, rinsed
- 1 onion, finely chopped
- 2 cloves garlic, minced
- 1 tablespoon curry powder
- 1 teaspoon ground cumin
- 1 teaspoon ground coriander
- ½ teaspoon turmeric
- 1 can coconut milk
- Salt and pepper, to taste
- Chopped fresh cilantro (for garnish)
- Cooked rice (for serving)

Preparation:

1. Heat olive oil in a large skillet or pot over medium heat. Add chopped onion and minced garlic, and cook until softened.

2. Stir in curry powder, ground cumin, ground coriander, and turmeric, and cook for 1 minute until fragrant.

3. Add diced sweet potatoes, rinsed lentils, and coconut milk to the skillet, stirring to combine.

4. Cover and simmer curry for 25-30 minutes, stirring occasionally, until sweet potatoes are tender and lentils are cooked.

5. Season with salt and pepper to make it tasty.

6. Serve hot over cooked rice, garnished with chopped fresh cilantro.

Nutritional Value (per serving):

- Calories: 300
- Protein: 10g
- Carbohydrates: 40g

- Fat: 10g
- Fiber: 12g

Cooking Time: 30 minutes

Notes:

_____

_____

_____

_____

_____

_____

Progress Report:

_____

_____

_____

_____

_____

_____

CHAPTER 5

Snack Recipes

1. Trail Mix with Nuts and Dried Fruit

Ingredients:

- 1 cup of mixed nuts (like cashews, walnuts, almonds etc.)

- ½ cup dried fruit (raisins, cranberries, apricots, etc.)

- ¼ cup seeds (pumpkin seeds, sunflower seeds, etc.)

Preparation:

1. In a bowl, combine mixed nuts, dried fruit, and seeds.

2. Toss gently to mix.

3. Store in an airtight container for snacking.

Nutritional Value (per serving):

- Calories: 200

- Protein: 5g

- Carbohydrates: 15g

- Fat: 12g

- Fiber: 3g

Notes:

_____

_____

_____

_____

_____

_____

Progress Report:

_____

_____

_____

_____

_____

_____

2. Edamame with Sea Salt

- 1 cup edamame (fresh or frozen)
- Sea salt, to taste

1. If you're using frozen edamame, cook it as directed on the package. If using fresh, steam or boil until tender.
2. Sprinkle with sea salt before serving.

- Calories: 100
- Protein: 9g
- Carbohydrates: 8g
- Fat: 4g
- Fiber: 4g

Cooking Time: 5-10 minutes

Notes:

_____

_____

_____

_____

_____

_____

Progress Report:

_____

_____

_____

_____

_____

_____

3. Roasted Chickpeas

Ingredients:

- 1 can chickpeas, drained and rinsed

- 1 tablespoon olive oil

- 1 teaspoon paprika

- ½ teaspoon garlic powder

- Salt and pepper, to taste

Preparation:

1. Preheat oven to 400°F (200°C).

2. Pat chickpeas dry with a paper towel and place on a baking sheet.

3. Drizzle with olive oil and sprinkle with paprika, garlic powder, salt, and pepper.

4. Toss to coat evenly.

5. Roast in the preheated oven for 25-30 minutes, until crispy.

6. Let cool before serving.

Nutritional Value (per serving):

- Calories: 150

- Protein: 6g

- Carbohydrates: 20g

- Fat: 5g

- Fiber: 6g

Cooking Time: 25-30 minutes

Notes:

_____

_____

_____

_____

_____

_____

Progress Report:

_____

_____

_____

_____

_____

_____

4. Cucumber and Avocado Sushi Rolls

Ingredients:

- 2 sheets nori seaweed
- ½ cucumber, julienned
- 1 avocado, sliced
- Cooked sushi rice
- Soy sauce and wasabi (for serving)

Preparation:

1. On a bamboo sushi mat, spread a sheet of nori seaweed.

2. Spread a thin layer of cooked sushi rice over the nori, leaving a small border at the top.

3. Arrange cucumber and avocado slices in a line along the bottom edge of the nori.

4. Roll the sushi tightly using the bamboo mat, sealing the edge with water.

5. Slice into bite-sized pieces using a sharp knife.

6. Serve with soy sauce and wasabi.

Nutritional Value (per serving):

- Calories: 200

- Protein: 5g

- Carbohydrates: 30g

- Fat: 8g

- Fiber: 5g

Cooking Time: 20 minutes

Notes:

_____

_____

_____

_____

_____

_____

Progress Report:

_____

_____

_____

_____

_____

_____

5. Carrot and Hummus Pinwheels

Ingredients:

- 2 large carrots, peeled
- ½ cup hummus
- Salt and pepper, to taste

Preparation:

1. Use a vegetable peeler to slice the carrots into thin strips.
2. Spread hummus evenly over each carrot strip.
3. Season with salt and pepper.
4. Roll up the carrot strips tightly.
5. Secure with toothpicks if necessary.

Nutritional Value (per serving):

- Calories: 100
- Protein: 3g

- Carbohydrates: 15g
- Fat: 4g
- Fiber: 5g

Notes:

_____

_____

_____

_____

_____

_____

Progress Report:

_____

_____

_____

_____

_____

_____

6. Baked Garlic Herb Turkey Meatballs

Ingredients:

- 1 pound ground turkey
- ¼ cup breadcrumbs
- 1 egg
- 2 cloves garlic, minced
- 2 tablespoons of chopped fresh herbs (like thyme, rosemary, or parsley)
- Salt and pepper, to taste

Preparation:

1. Preheat oven to 375°F (190°C).
2. In a bowl, combine ground turkey, breadcrumbs, egg, minced garlic, chopped fresh herbs, salt, and pepper.
3. Shape mixture into small meatballs and place on a baking sheet lined with parchment paper.

4. Bake in the preheated oven for 20-25 minutes, until cooked through.

5. Let cool before serving.

Nutritional Value (per serving):

- Calories: 150

- Protein: 20g

- Carbohydrates: 5g

- Fat: 6g

- Fiber: 1g

Cooking Time: 20-25 minutes

Notes:

_____

_____

_____

_____

_____

_____

Progress Report:

_____

_____

_____

_____

_____

_____

7. Grilled Herb Marinated Quail

Ingredients:

- 4 quail
- 2 tablespoons olive oil
- 2 cloves garlic, minced
- 1 tablespoon of chopped fresh herbs (like rosemary, sage or thyme)
- Salt and pepper, to taste

Preparation:

1. In a bowl, whisk together olive oil, minced garlic, chopped fresh herbs, salt, and pepper.

2. Place quail in a shallow dish and pour the marinade over them, making sure they are evenly coated. For a minimum of half an hour and a maximum of four hours, marinate in the refrigerator.

3. Preheat grill to medium-high heat. Take out the quail from the marinade and throw away any extra marinade.

4. Grill quail for 4-5 minutes per side, or until cooked through.

5. Before serving, take off of the grill and give it a few minutes to rest.

Nutritional Value (per serving):

- Calories: 200
- Protein: 25g
- Carbohydrates: 0g
- Fat: 10g
- Fiber: 0g

Cooking Time: 10 minutes

Notes:

_____

_____

_____

_____

_____

_____

Progress Report:

_____

_____

_____

_____

_____

_____

8. Baked Quail with Apricot Glaze

Ingredients:

- 4 quail
- ¼ cup apricot preserves
- 1 tablespoon Dijon mustard
- 1 tablespoon balsamic vinegar
- Salt and pepper, to taste

Preparation:

1. Preheat oven to 375°F (190°C). Line a baking dish with parchment paper.

2. In a small bowl, whisk together apricot preserves, Dijon mustard, balsamic vinegar, salt, and pepper.

3. Place quail in the prepared baking dish and brush with apricot glaze, covering them evenly.

4. Bake in the preheated oven for 20-25 minutes, until cooked through, basting occasionally with glaze.

5. Remove from oven and let rest for a few minutes before serving.

Nutritional Value (per serving):

- Calories: 250
- Protein: 20g
- Carbohydrates: 15g
- Fat: 10g
- Fiber: 0g

Cooking Time: 25 minutes

Notes:

_____

_____

_____

_____

_____

_____

Progress Report:

_____

_____

_____

_____

_____

_____

9. Quail Stuffed with Quinoa and Vegetables

Ingredients:

- 4 quail

- 1 cup cooked quinoa

- ½ cup diced Veggies (like bell peppers, onions, and mushrooms)

- 2 cloves garlic, minced

- 1 tablespoon olive oil

- Salt and pepper, to taste

Preparation:

1. Preheat oven to 375°F (190°C). Ensure you line a baking dish with parchment paper.

2. Heat the olive oil in a pan over medium heat. Add minced garlic and diced vegetables, and cook until softened.

3. Stir in cooked quinoa and season with salt and pepper to taste.

4. Stuff each quail with quinoa and vegetable mixture.

5. Place quail in the prepared baking dish and bake in the preheated oven for 20-25 minutes, until cooked through.

6. Remove from oven and let rest for a few minutes before serving.

Nutritional Value (per serving):

- Calories: 300

- Protein: 25g

- Carbohydrates: 20g

- Fat: 12g

- Fiber: 3g

Cooking Time: 25 minutes

Notes:

_____

_____

_____

_____

_____

_____

Progress Report:

_____

_____

_____

_____

_____

_____

10. Braised Beef with Tomatoes and Herbs

Ingredients:

- 1 pound beef stew meat

- 1 onion, chopped

- 2 cloves garlic, minced

- 1 can diced tomatoes

- 1 cup beef broth

- 1 tablespoon chopped fresh herbs (such as rosemary, thyme, or oregano)

- Salt and pepper, to taste

Preparation:

1. In a large skillet or pot, heat olive oil over medium heat. Add chopped onion and minced garlic, and cook until softened.

2. Add beef stew meat to the skillet and cook until browned on all sides.

3. Stir in diced tomatoes, beef broth, chopped fresh herbs, salt, and pepper.

4. Bring to a simmer, then reduce heat to low and cover. Let simmer for 1-2 hours, stirring occasionally, until beef is tender.

5. Serve hot.

Nutritional Value (per serving):

- Calories: 250

- Protein: 25g

- Carbohydrates: 10g

- Fat: 12g

- Fiber: 3g

Cooking Time: 2 hours

Notes:

_____

_____

_____

_____

_____

_____

Progress Report:

_____

_____

_____

_____

_____

_____

30 Day Meal Plan

Week 1

Day 1:

Breakfast: Creamy Oatmeal with Fresh Berries

Lunch: Baked Lemon Herb Salmon

Dinner: Lemon Herb Grilled Chicken Breast

Snack: Trail Mix with Nuts and Dried Fruit

Day 2:

Breakfast: Scrambled Eggs with Spinach and Feta

Lunch: Grilled Shrimp Skewers

Dinner: Herb Crusted Chicken Thighs

Snack: Edamame with Sea Salt

Day 3:

Breakfast: Banana Walnut Pancakes

Lunch: Baked Cod with Tomato and Basil

Dinner: Honey Mustard Glazed Turkey Breast

Snack: Roasted Chickpeas

Day 4:

Breakfast: Greek Yogurt Parfait

Lunch: Lemon Garlic Butter Scallops

Dinner: Zucchini Noodles with Pesto

Snack: Cucumber and Avocado Sushi Rolls

Day 5:

Breakfast: Apple Cinnamon Quinoa Porridge

Lunch: Salmon and Asparagus Foil Packet

Dinner: Creamy Mushroom Risotto

Snack: Carrot and Hummus Pinwheels

Day 6:

Breakfast: Avocado Toast with Poached Eggs

Lunch: Lime Cilantro Shrimp Tacos

Dinner: Baked Eggplant Parmesan

Snack: Baked Garlic Herb Turkey Meatballs

Day 7:

Breakfast: Sweet Potato Hash with Turkey Sausage

Lunch: Baked Teriyaki Salmon

Dinner: Cauliflower and Broccoli Bake

Snack: Grilled Herb Marinated Quail

Week 2

Breakfast: Blueberry Chia Pudding

Lunch: Broiled Lemon Pepper Haddock

Dinner: Eggplant and Chickpea Curry

Snack: Baked Quail with Apricot Glaze

Breakfast: Cottage Cheese and Fruit Bowl

Lunch: Shrimp and Vegetable Stir Fry

Dinner: Ratatouille

Snack: Quail Stuffed with Quinoa and Vegetables

Breakfast: Zucchini and Carrot Fritters

Lunch: Baked Garlic Herb Mussels

Dinner: Sweet Potato and Lentil Curry

Snack: Braised Beef with Tomatoes and Herbs

Day 11:

Breakfast: Avocado Toast with Poached Eggs

Lunch: Lime Cilantro Shrimp Tacos

Dinner: Baked Eggplant Parmesan

Snack: Baked Garlic Herb Turkey Meatballs

Day 12:

Breakfast: Sweet Potato Hash with Turkey Sausage

Lunch: Baked Teriyaki Salmon

Dinner: Cauliflower and Broccoli Bake

Snack: Grilled Herb Marinated Quail

Day 13:

Breakfast: Blueberry Chia Pudding

Lunch: Broiled Lemon Pepper Haddock

Dinner: Eggplant and Chickpea Curry

Snack: Baked Quail with Apricot Glaze

Day 14:

Breakfast: Cottage Cheese and Fruit Bowl

Lunch: Shrimp and Vegetable Stir Fry

Dinner: Ratatouille

Snack: Quail Stuffed with Quinoa and Vegetables

Week 3

Breakfast: Zucchini and Carrot Fritters

Lunch: Baked Garlic Herb Mussels

Dinner: Sweet Potato and Lentil Curry

Snack: Braised Beef with Tomatoes and Herbs

Breakfast: Creamy Oatmeal with Fresh Berries

Lunch: Baked Lemon Herb Salmon

Dinner: Lemon Herb Grilled Chicken Breast

Snack: Trail Mix with Nuts and Dried Fruit

Breakfast: Scrambled Eggs with Spinach and Feta

Lunch: Grilled Shrimp Skewers

Dinner: Herb Crusted Chicken Thighs

Snack: Edamame with Sea Salt

Day 18:

Breakfast: Banana Walnut Pancakes

Lunch: Baked Cod with Tomato and Basil

Dinner: Honey Mustard Glazed Turkey Breast

Snack: Roasted Chickpeas

Day 19:

Breakfast: Greek Yogurt Parfait

Lunch: Lemon Garlic Butter Scallops

Dinner: Zucchini Noodles with Pesto

Snack: Cucumber and Avocado Sushi Rolls

Day 20:

Breakfast: Apple Cinnamon Quinoa Porridge

Lunch: Salmon and Asparagus Foil Packet

Dinner: Creamy Mushroom Risotto

Snack: Carrot and Hummus Pinwheels

Day 21:

Breakfast: Creamy Oatmeal with Fresh Berries

Lunch: Baked Lemon Herb Salmon

Dinner: Lemon Herb Grilled Chicken Breast

Snack: Trail Mix with Nuts and Dried Fruit

Week 4

Day 22:

Breakfast: Scrambled Eggs with Spinach and Feta

Lunch: Grilled Shrimp Skewers

Dinner: Herb Crusted Chicken Thighs

Snack: Edamame with Sea Salt

Day 23:

Breakfast: Banana Walnut Pancakes

Lunch: Baked Cod with Tomato and Basil

Dinner: Honey Mustard Glazed Turkey Breast

Snack: Roasted Chickpeas

Day 24:

Breakfast: Greek Yogurt Parfait

Lunch: Lemon Garlic Butter Scallops

Dinner: Zucchini Noodles with Pesto

Snack: Cucumber and Avocado Sushi Rolls

Day 25:

Breakfast: Apple Cinnamon Quinoa Porridge

Lunch: Salmon and Asparagus Foil Packet

Dinner: Creamy Mushroom Risotto

Snack: Carrot and Hummus Pinwheels

Day 26:

Breakfast: Avocado Toast with Poached Eggs

Lunch: Lime Cilantro Shrimp Tacos

Dinner: Baked Eggplant Parmesan

Snack: Baked Garlic Herb Turkey Meatballs

Day 27:

Breakfast: Sweet Potato Hash with Turkey Sausage

Lunch: Baked Teriyaki Salmon

Dinner: Cauliflower and Broccoli Bake

Snack: Grilled Herb Marinated Quail

Day 28:

Breakfast: Blueberry Chia Pudding

Lunch: Broiled Lemon Pepper Haddock

Dinner: Eggplant and Chickpea Curry

Snack: Baked Quail with Apricot Glaze

Day 29:

Breakfast: Cottage Cheese and Fruit Bowl

Lunch: Shrimp and Vegetable Stir Fry

Dinner: Ratatouille

Snack: Quail Stuffed with Quinoa and Vegetables

Day 30:

Breakfast: Zucchini and Carrot Fritters

Lunch: Baked Garlic Herb Mussels

Dinner: Sweet Potato and Lentil Curry

Snack: Braised Beef with Tomatoes and Herbs

CONCLUSION

Finally, I would like to express my profound appreciation to you, my dear reader, for spending the time to look through this selection of recipes that are safe for gallbladders. It is impressive that you are dedicated to finding answers to your health issues, and I sincerely hope that this book has given you useful information and useful recipes to help you on your journey.

I hope you have the utmost success incorporating these recipes into your everyday routine. I hope that cooking and eating these filling meals will bring you happiness and ease as you go through them.

I sincerely hope that this book will be your last resource for any problems pertaining to the health of your gallbladder. You are taking proactive measures to maximize your well-being and recover control over your health by including these expertly prepared recipes into your diet.

Never forget that even the smallest adjustment you make to your lifestyle can have a big impact. Have faith in the process, practice self-compassion, and don't be afraid to seek support when you need it.

Cheers to your continued well-being and vigor. I hope the journey bring you plenty of energy, health, and the satisfaction of enjoying tasty, gallbladder-friendly meals.

My Little Request

Dear Reader,

Thanks for your purchase, hope you enjoyed reading.

Could you please take a few seconds to leave a positive feedback on this book?

It'll help reach more people and we can collectively live healthier lives.

Thank you.

BONUS: MEAL PLANNER JOURNAL

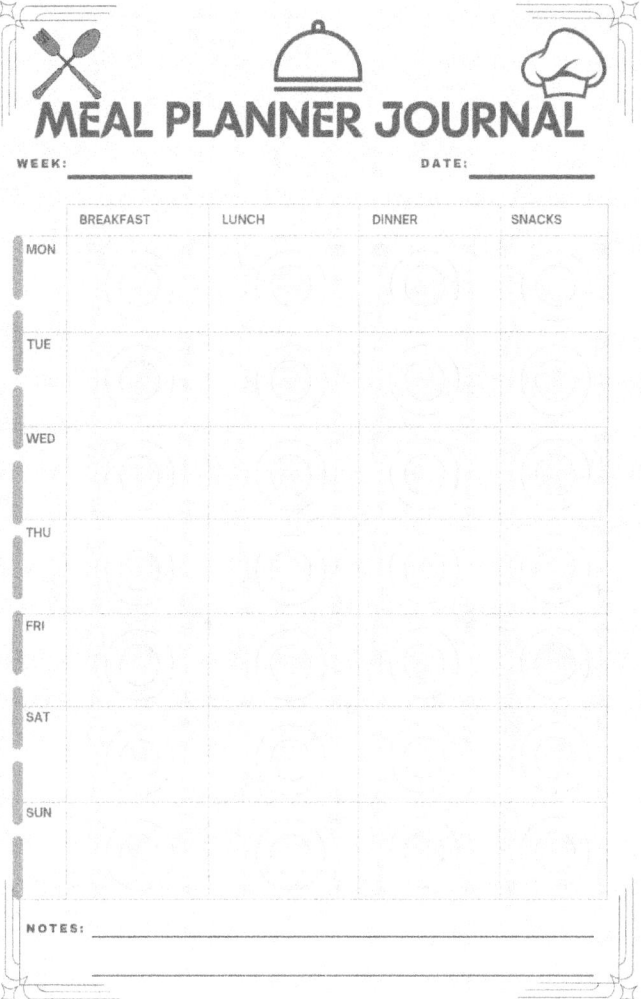

MEAL PLANNER JOURNAL

WEEK: _____   DATE: _____

	BREAKFAST	LUNCH	DINNER	SNACKS
MON				
TUE				
WED				
THU				
FRI				
SAT				
SUN				

NOTES: _____

_____

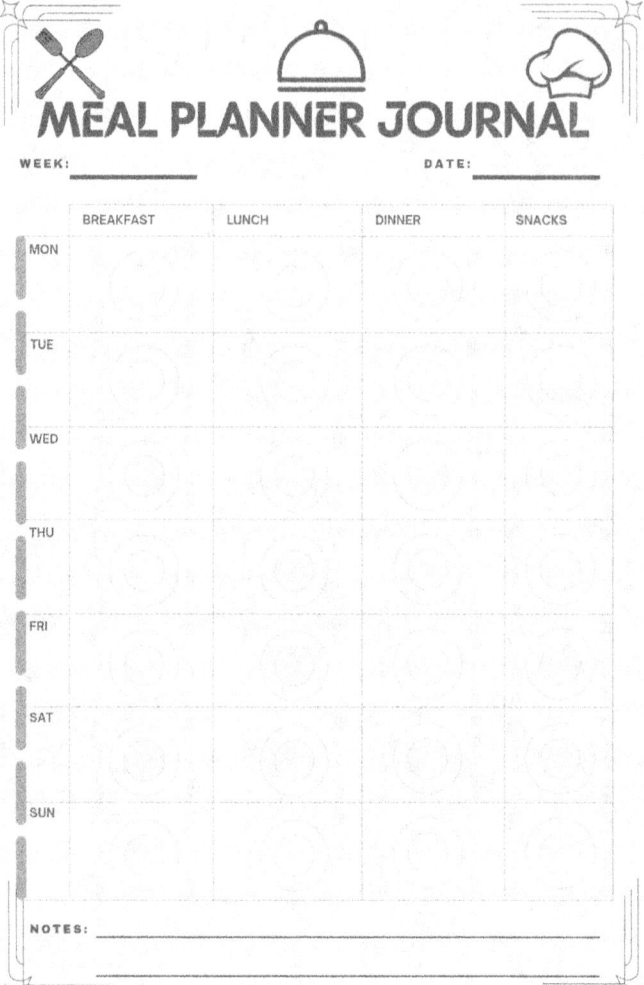

MEAL PLANNER JOURNAL

WEEK: _____   DATE: _____

	BREAKFAST	LUNCH	DINNER	SNACKS
MON				
TUE				
WED				
THU				
FRI				
SAT				
SUN				

NOTES: _____

_____

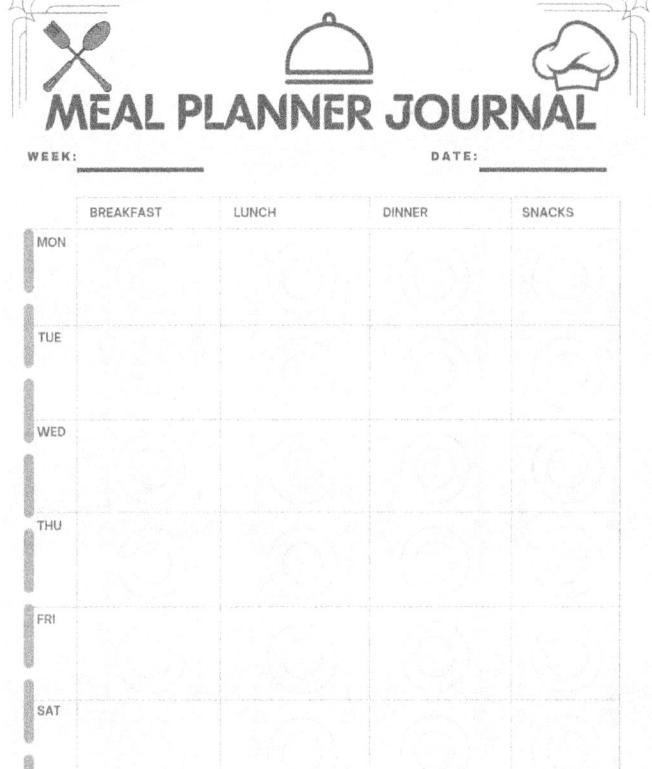

MEAL PLANNER JOURNAL

WEEK: _____   DATE: _____

	BREAKFAST	LUNCH	DINNER	SNACKS
MON				
TUE				
WED				
THU				
FRI				
SAT				
SUN				

NOTES: _____

_____

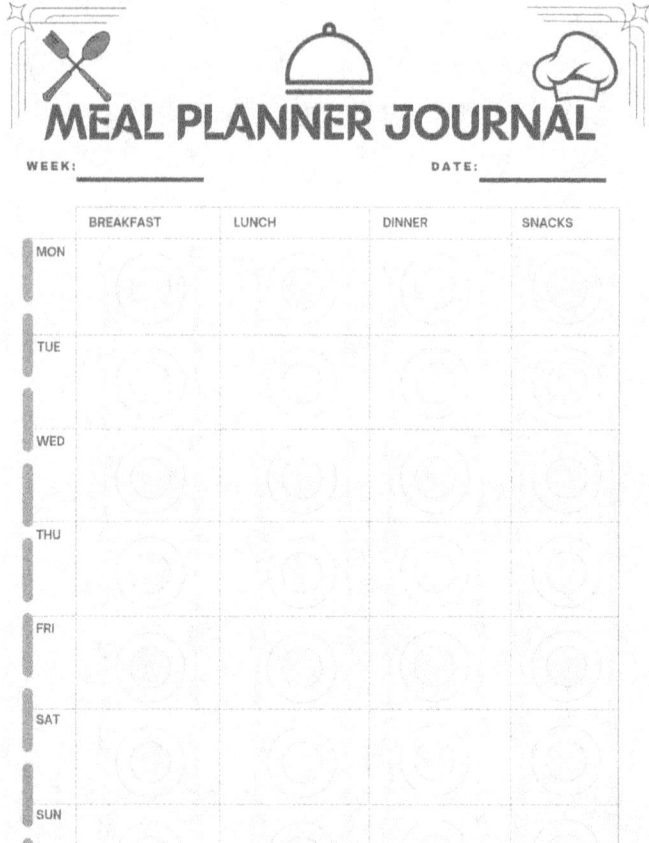

MEAL PLANNER JOURNAL

WEEK: _____   DATE: _____

	BREAKFAST	LUNCH	DINNER	SNACKS
MON				
TUE				
WED				
THU				
FRI				
SAT				
SUN				

NOTES: _____

_____

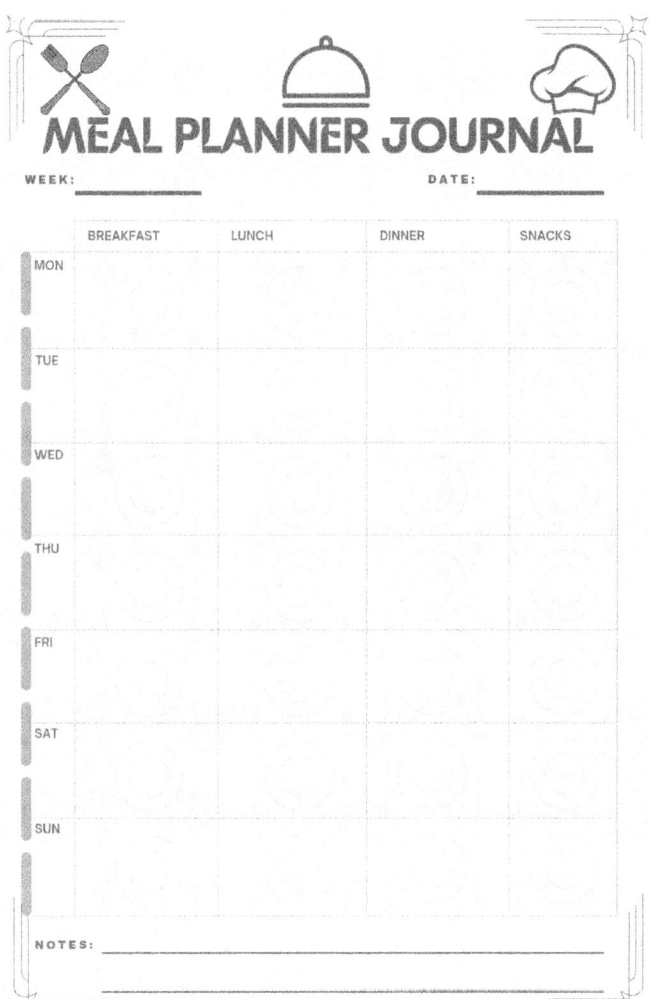

MEAL PLANNER JOURNAL

WEEK: _____   DATE: _____

	BREAKFAST	LUNCH	DINNER	SNACKS
MON				
TUE				
WED				
THU				
FRI				
SAT				
SUN				

NOTES: _____

_____

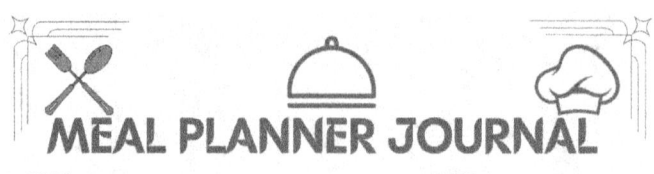

MEAL PLANNER JOURNAL

WEEK: _____   DATE: _____

	BREAKFAST	LUNCH	DINNER	SNACKS
MON				
TUE				
WED				
THU				
FRI				
SAT				
SUN				

NOTES: _____

_____

MEAL PLANNER JOURNAL

WEEK: _____   DATE: _____

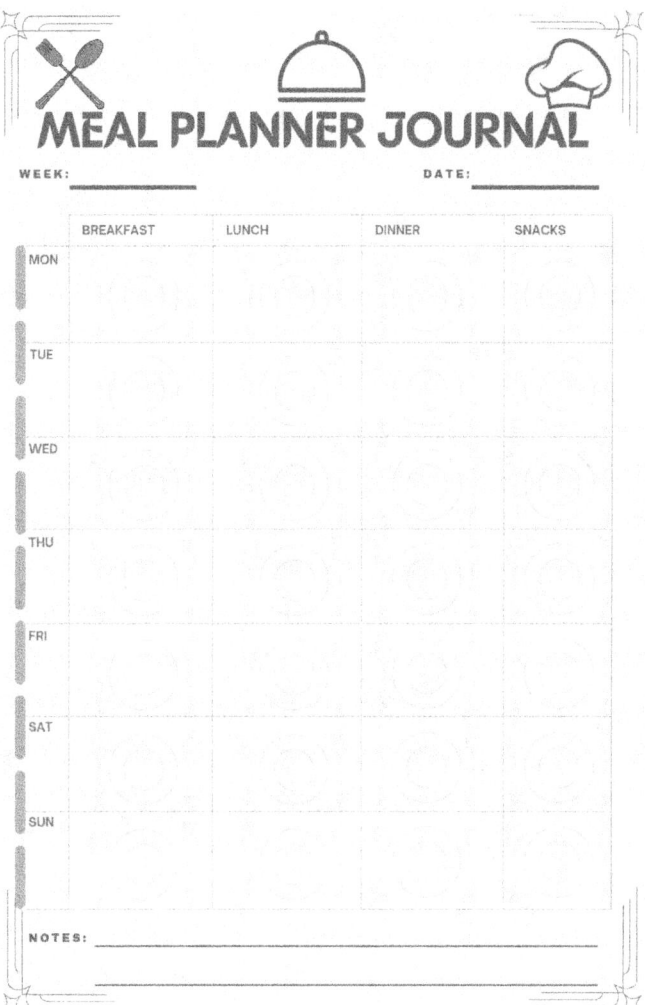

	BREAKFAST	LUNCH	DINNER	SNACKS
MON				
TUE				
WED				
THU				
FRI				
SAT				
SUN				

NOTES: _____

_____

MEAL PLANNER JOURNAL

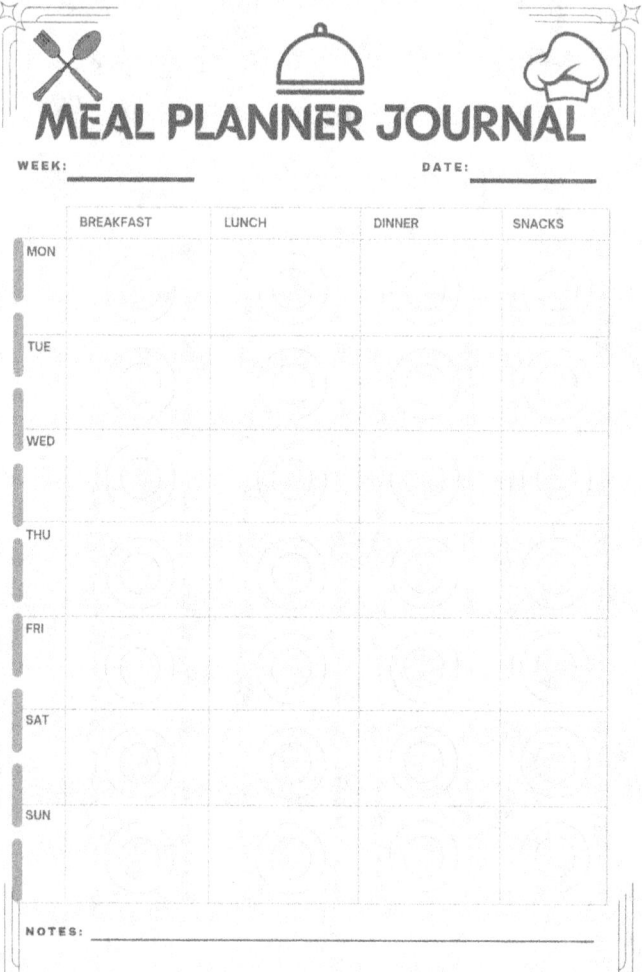

WEEK: _____   DATE: _____

	BREAKFAST	LUNCH	DINNER	SNACKS
MON				
TUE				
WED				
THU				
FRI				
SAT				
SUN				

NOTES: _____

_____

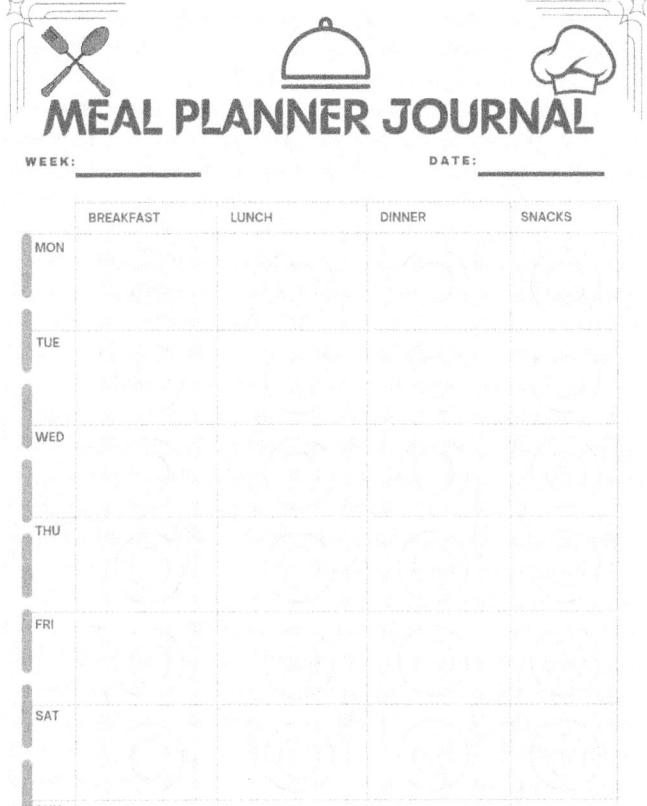

MEAL PLANNER JOURNAL

WEEK: _____   DATE: _____

	BREAKFAST	LUNCH	DINNER	SNACKS
MON				
TUE				
WED				
THU				
FRI				
SAT				
SUN				

NOTES: _____

_____

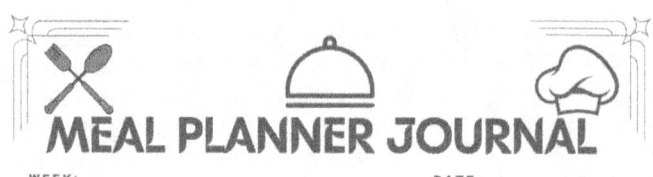

MEAL PLANNER JOURNAL

WEEK: _____   **DATE:** _____

	BREAKFAST	LUNCH	DINNER	SNACKS
MON				
TUE				
WED				
THU				
FRI				
SAT				
SUN				

NOTES: _____

_____

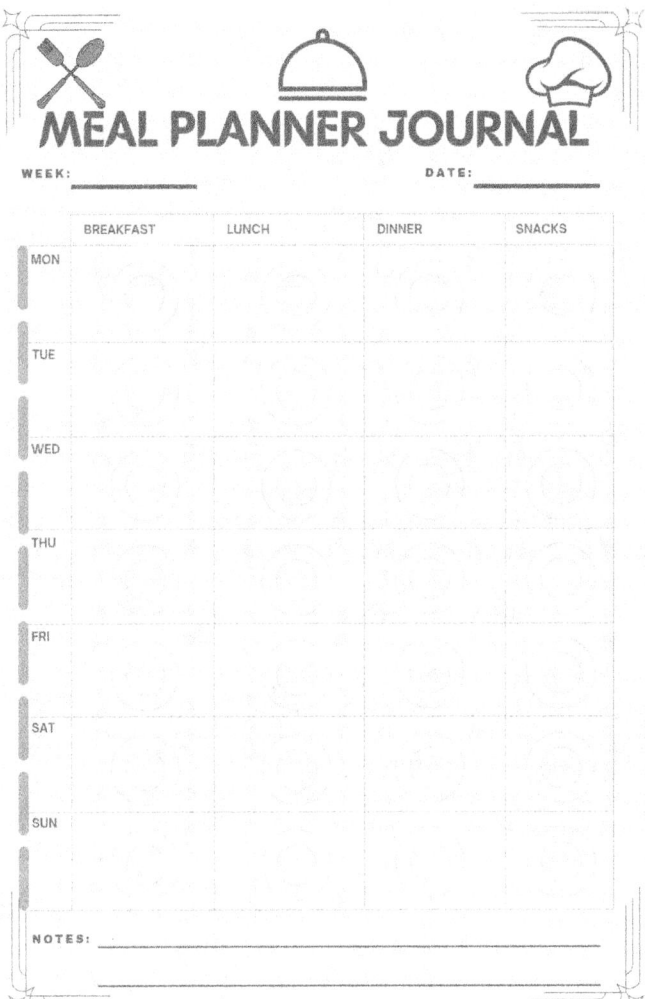

MEAL PLANNER JOURNAL

WEEK: _____   DATE: _____

	BREAKFAST	LUNCH	DINNER	SNACKS
MON				
TUE				
WED				
THU				
FRI				
SAT				
SUN				

NOTES: _____
_____

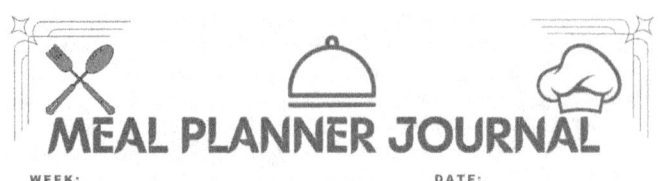

MEAL PLANNER JOURNAL

WEEK: _____   DATE: _____

	BREAKFAST	LUNCH	DINNER	SNACKS
MON				
TUE				
WED				
THU				
FRI				
SAT				
SUN				

NOTES: _____

_____

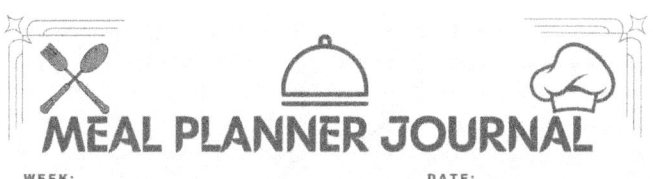

MEAL PLANNER JOURNAL

WEEK: _____ DATE: _____

	BREAKFAST	LUNCH	DINNER	SNACKS
MON				
TUE				
WED				
THU				
FRI				
SAT				
SUN				

NOTES: _____
_____

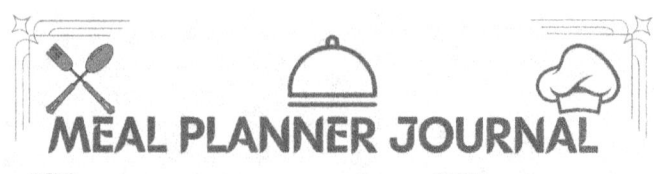

MEAL PLANNER JOURNAL

WEEK: _____   DATE: _____

	BREAKFAST	LUNCH	DINNER	SNACKS
MON				
TUE				
WED				
THU				
FRI				
SAT				
SUN				

NOTES: _____

_____

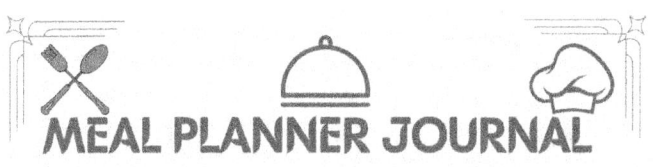

MEAL PLANNER JOURNAL

WEEK: _____   **DATE:** _____

	BREAKFAST	LUNCH	DINNER	SNACKS
MON				
TUE				
WED				
THU				
FRI				
SAT				
SUN				

NOTES: _____

_____

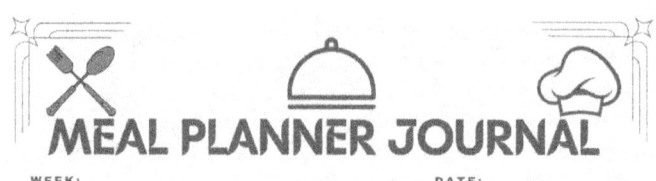

MEAL PLANNER JOURNAL

WEEK: _____   **DATE:** _____

	BREAKFAST	LUNCH	DINNER	SNACKS
MON				
TUE				
WED				
THU				
FRI				
SAT				
SUN				

NOTES: _____

_____

MEAL PLANNER JOURNAL

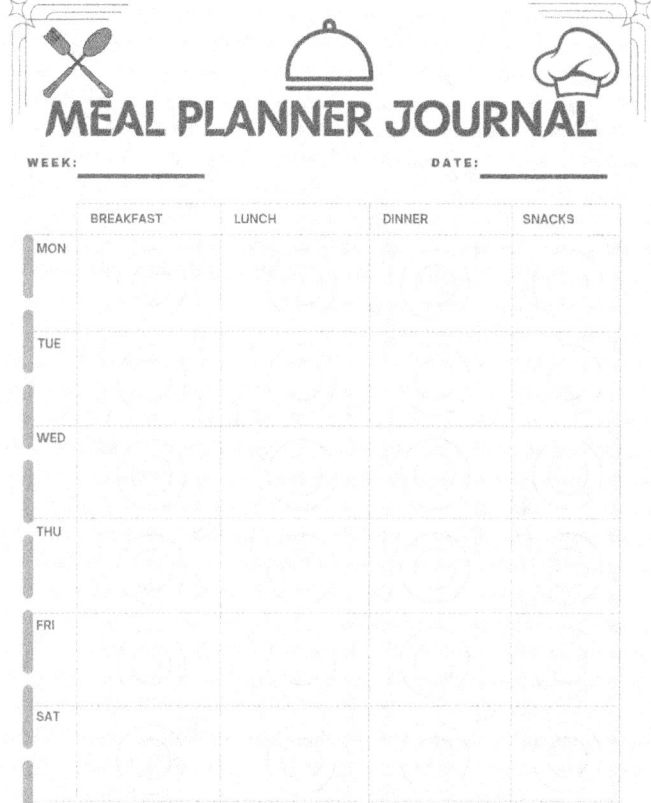

WEEK: _____   DATE: _____

	BREAKFAST	LUNCH	DINNER	SNACKS
MON				
TUE				
WED				
THU				
FRI				
SAT				
SUN				

NOTES: _____

_____

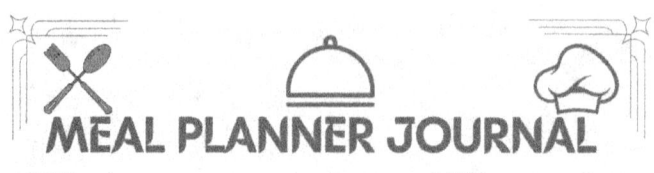

MEAL PLANNER JOURNAL

WEEK: _____   DATE: _____

	BREAKFAST	LUNCH	DINNER	SNACKS
MON				
TUE				
WED				
THU				
FRI				
SAT				
SUN				

NOTES: _____

_____

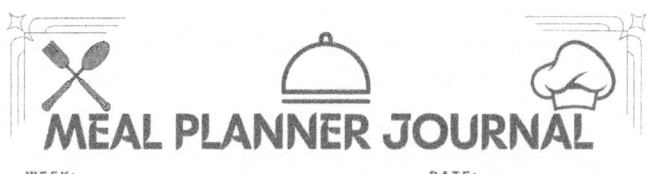

MEAL PLANNER JOURNAL

WEEK: _____   DATE: _____

	BREAKFAST	LUNCH	DINNER	SNACKS
MON				
TUE				
WED				
THU				
FRI				
SAT				
SUN				

NOTES: _____

_____

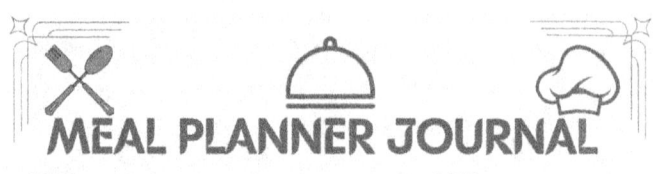

MEAL PLANNER JOURNAL

WEEK: _____   DATE: _____

	BREAKFAST	LUNCH	DINNER	SNACKS
MON				
TUE				
WED				
THU				
FRI				
SAT				
SUN				

NOTES: _____

_____

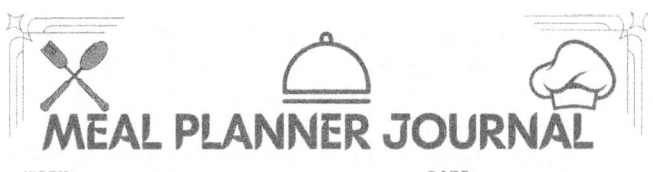

MEAL PLANNER JOURNAL

WEEK: _____   DATE: _____

	BREAKFAST	LUNCH	DINNER	SNACKS
MON				
TUE				
WED				
THU				
FRI				
SAT				
SUN				

NOTES: _____

_____

www.ingramcontent.com/pod-product-compliance
Lightning Source LLC
Chambersburg PA
CBHW071041290526
45795CB00004B/1252